RAY OF
FUCKEN
SUNSHINE

ADULT CUSSING COLORING BOOK FULL OF BEAUTIFUL PICTURES WITH CUSS WORDS TO COLOR TO RELIEVE STRESS-ANXIETY-DEPRESSION-SLEEPING ISSUES. ENJOY...

THIS SHIT BELONGS TO ME

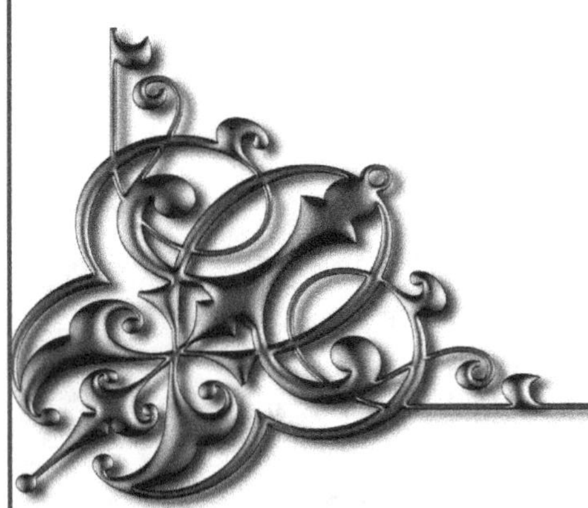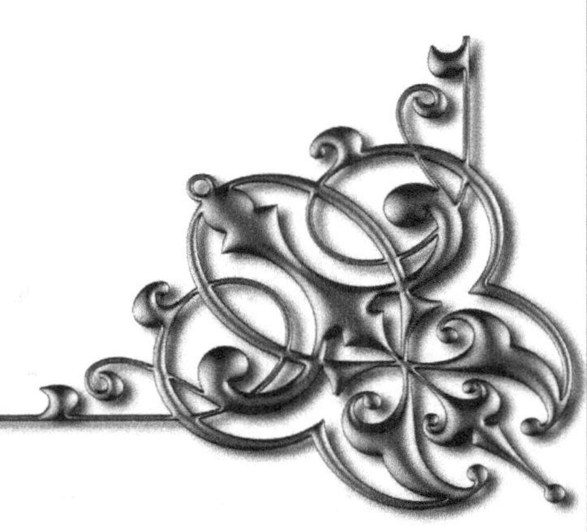

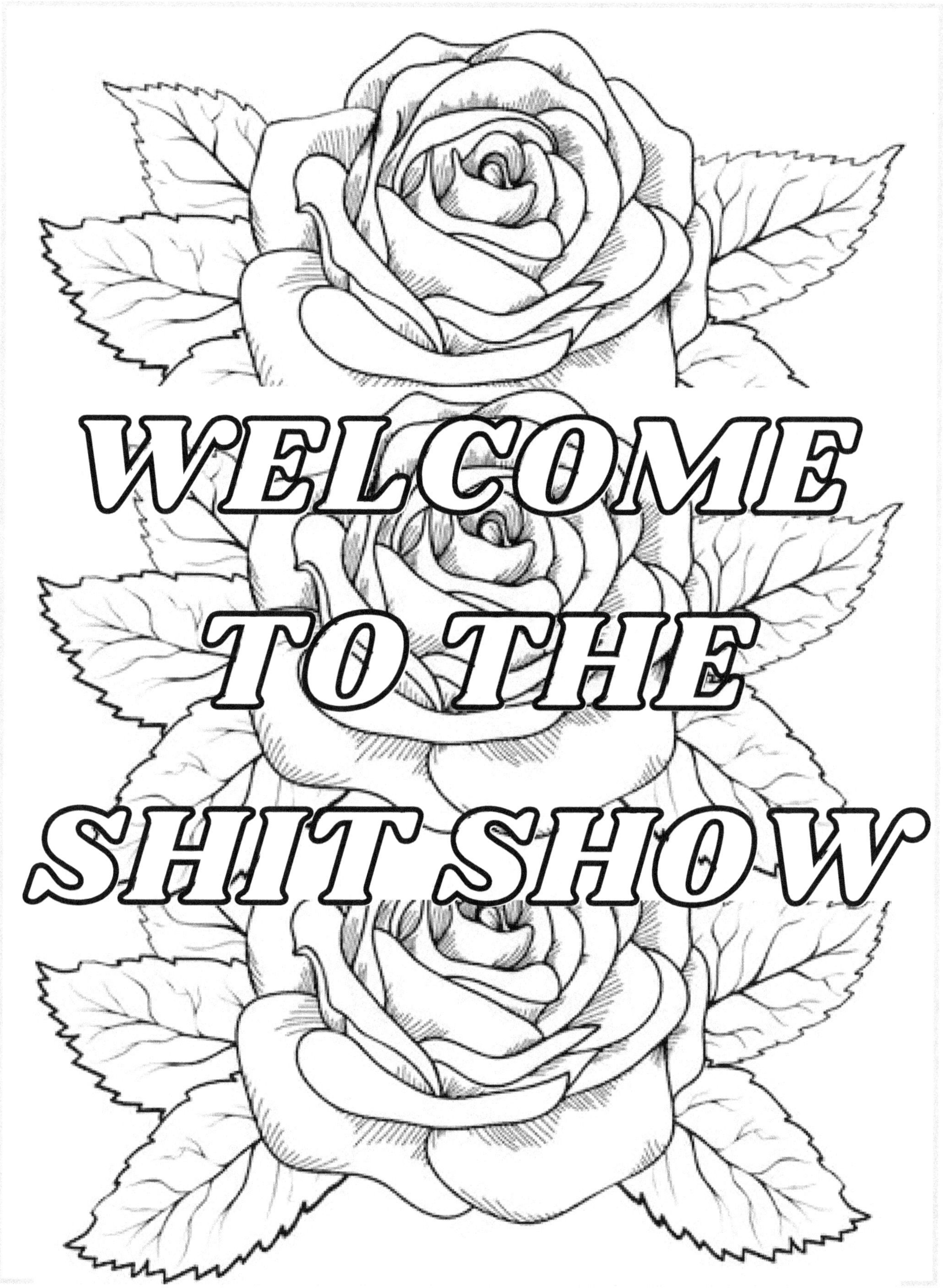

WELCOME TO THE SHIT SHOW

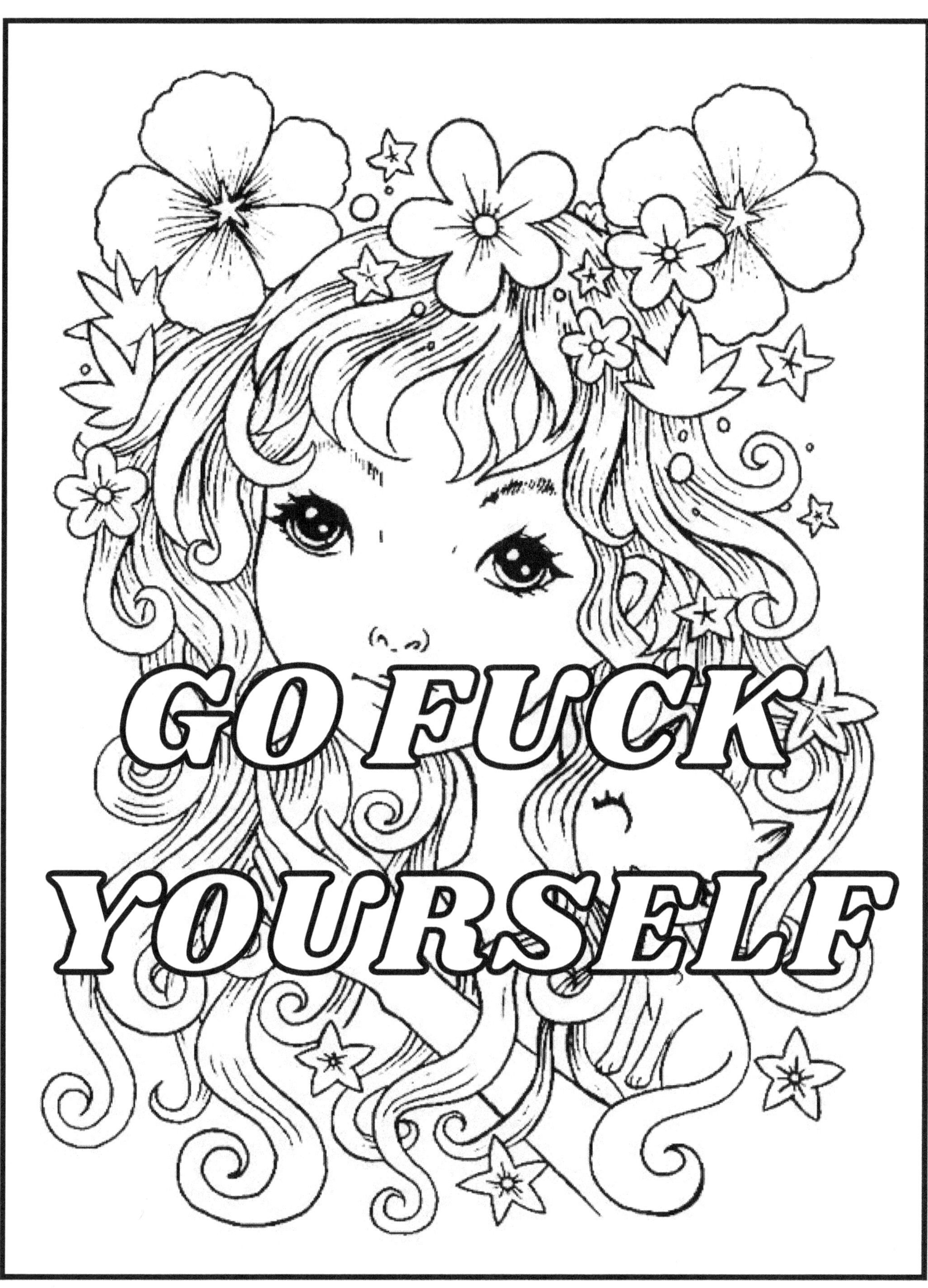
GO FUCK
YOURSELF

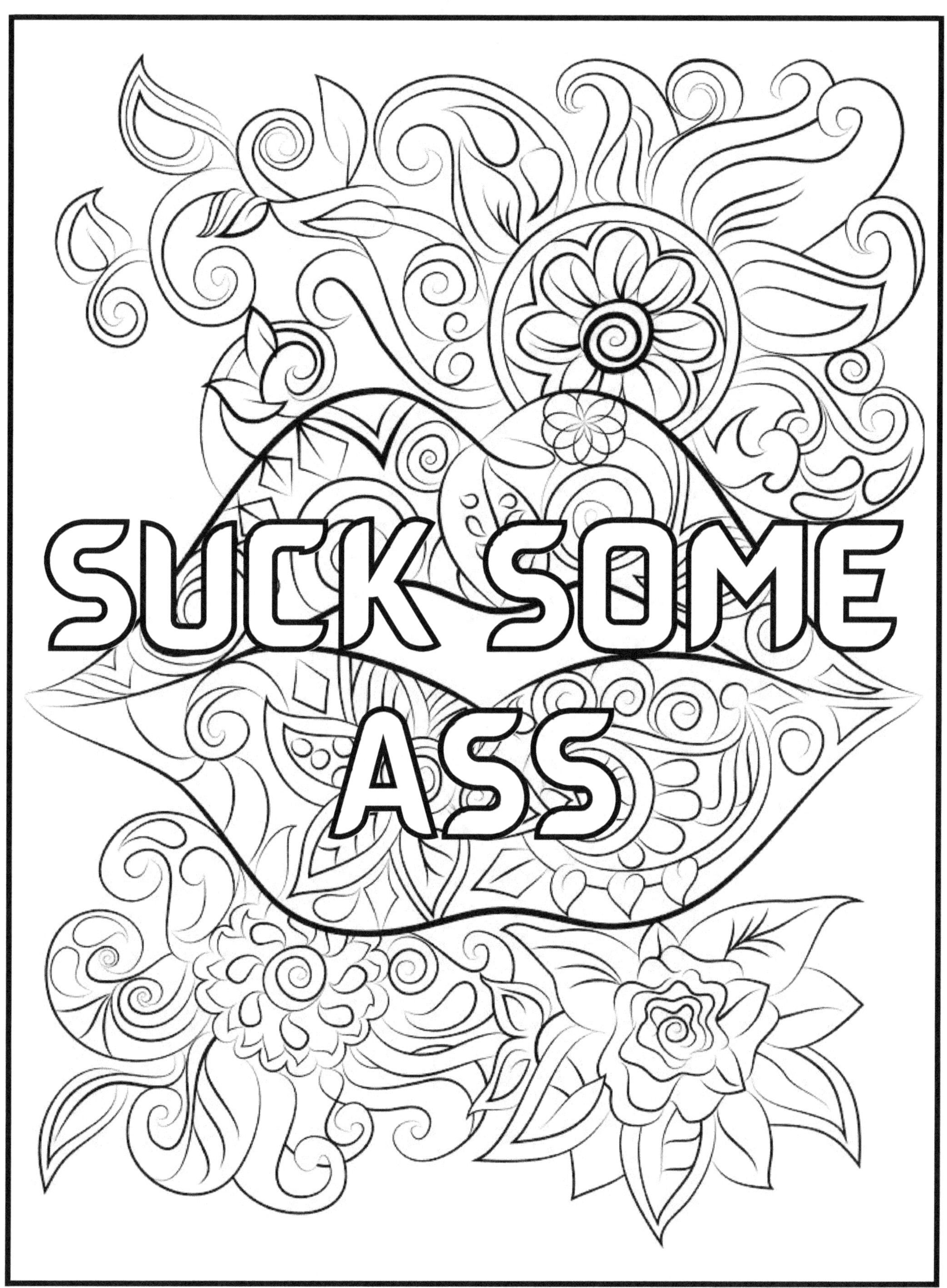

SUCK SOME
ASS

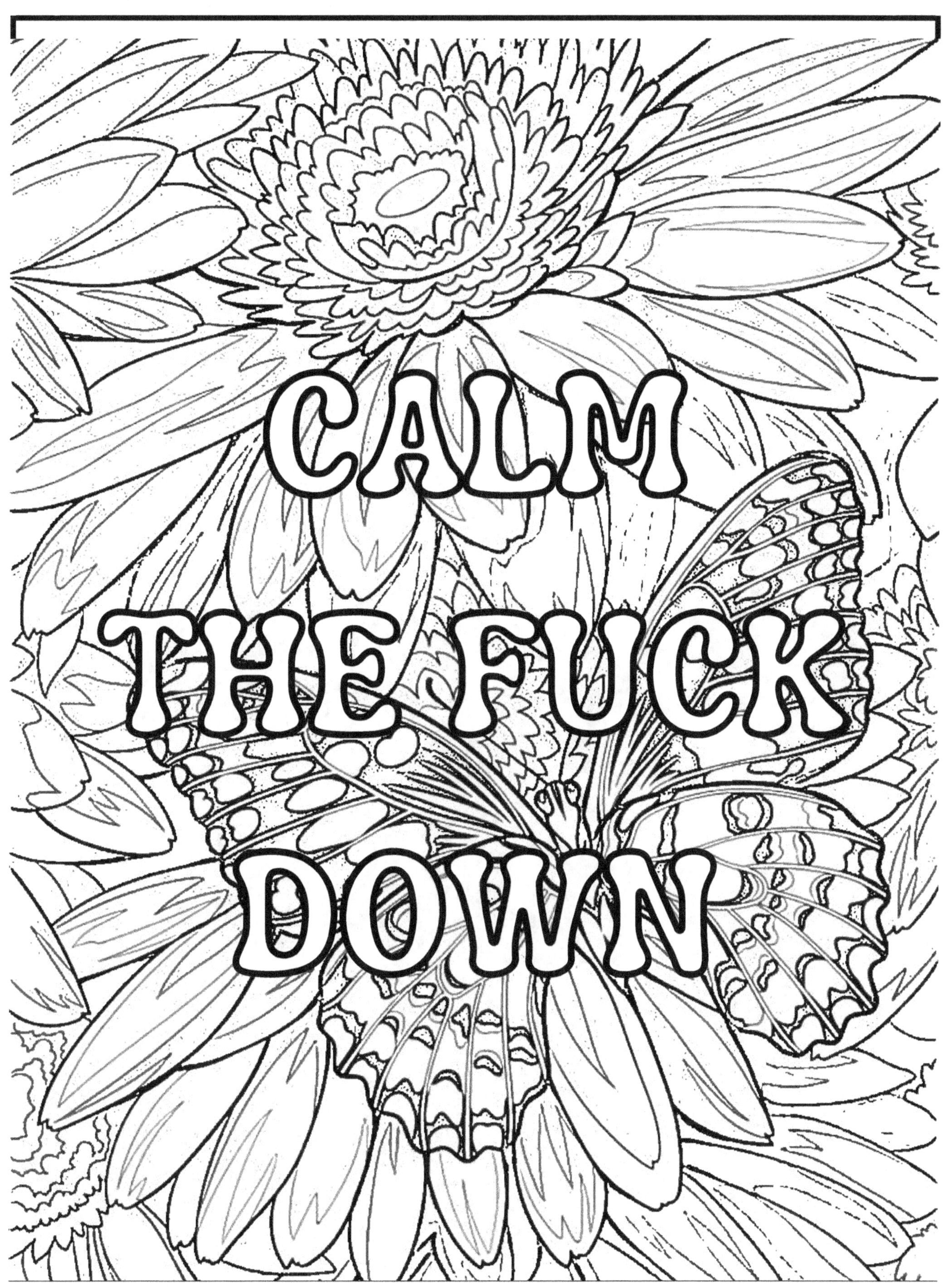
CALM
THE FUCK
DOWN

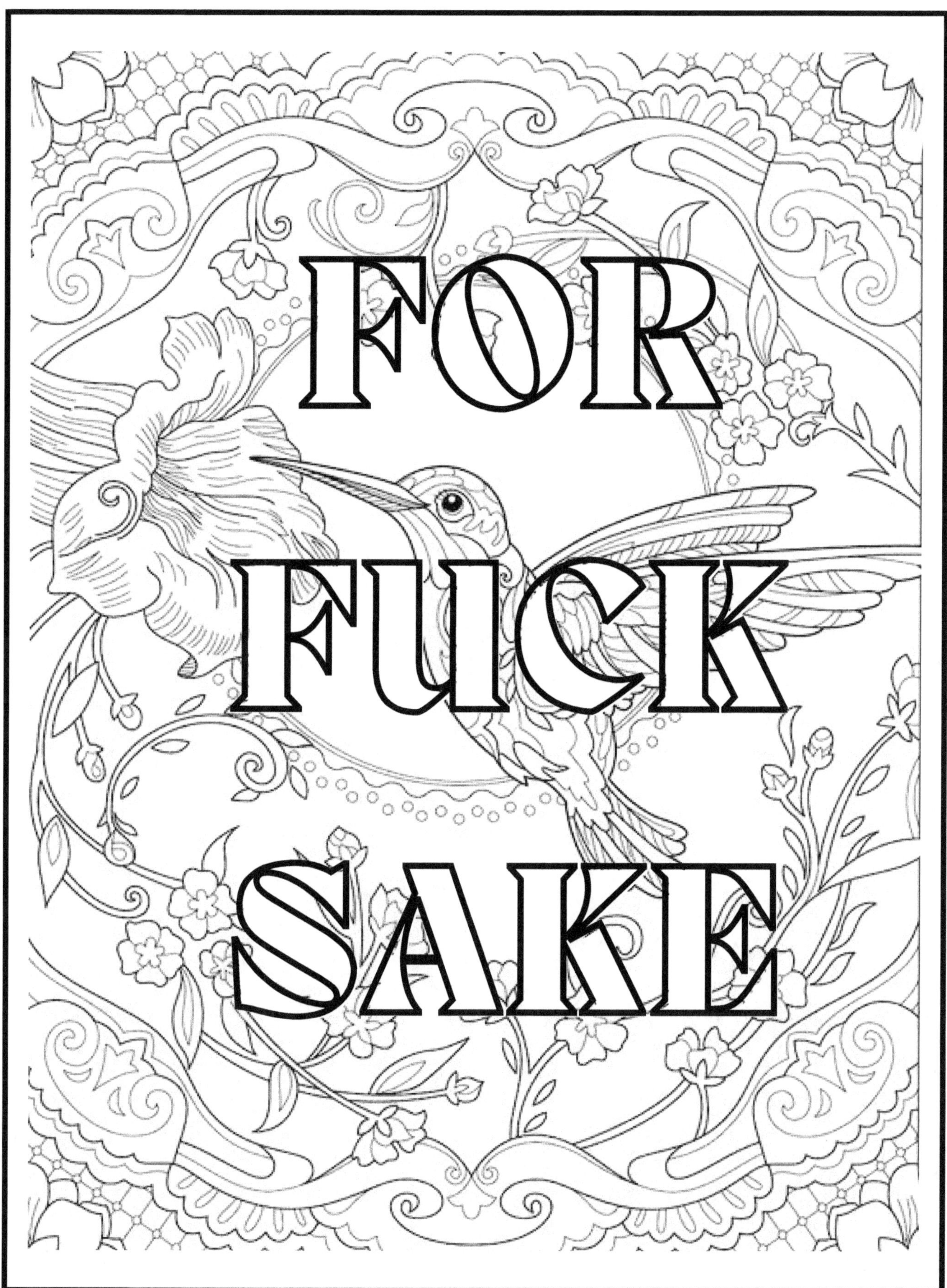

FOR
FUCK
SAKE

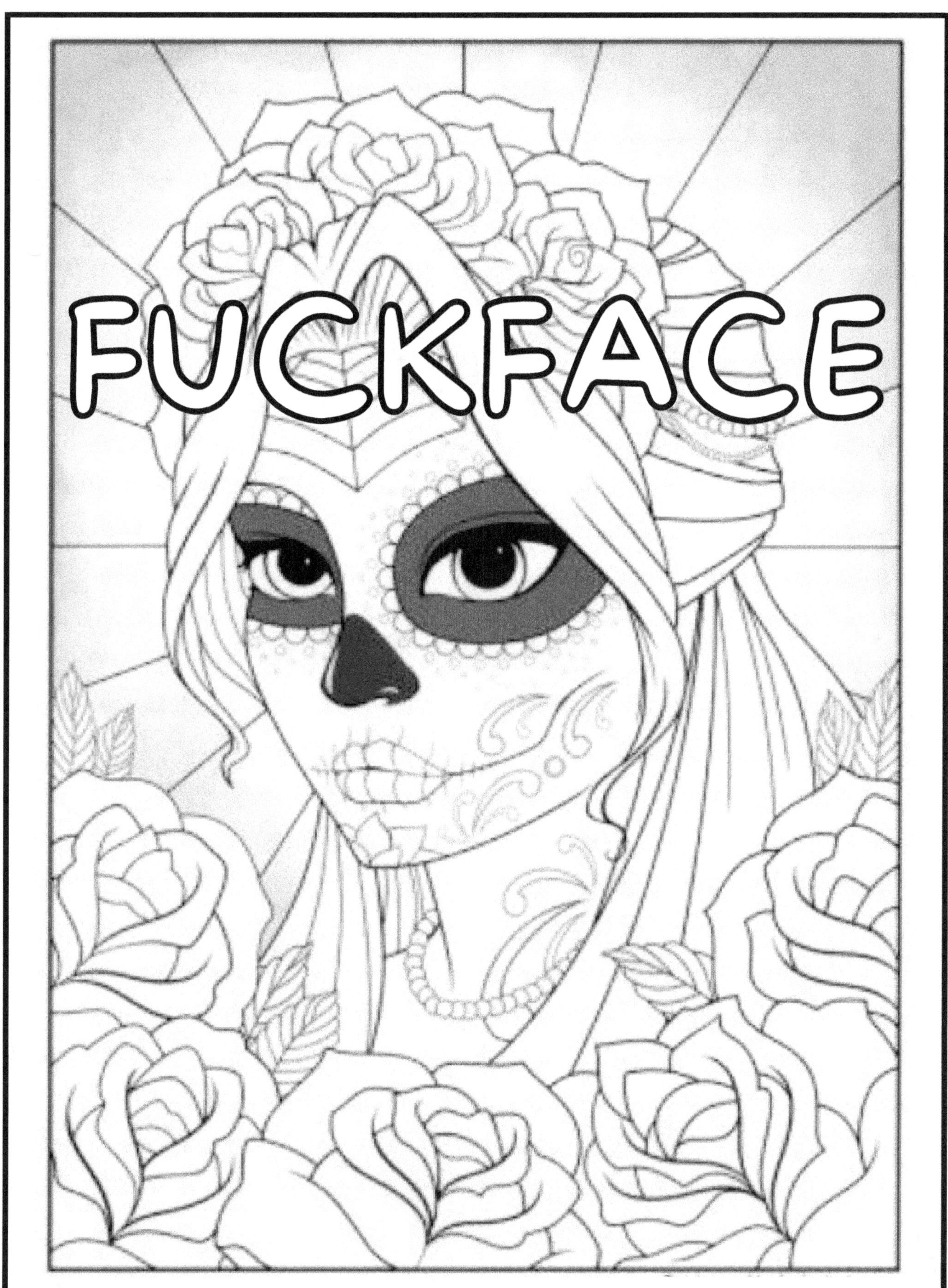
FUCKFACE

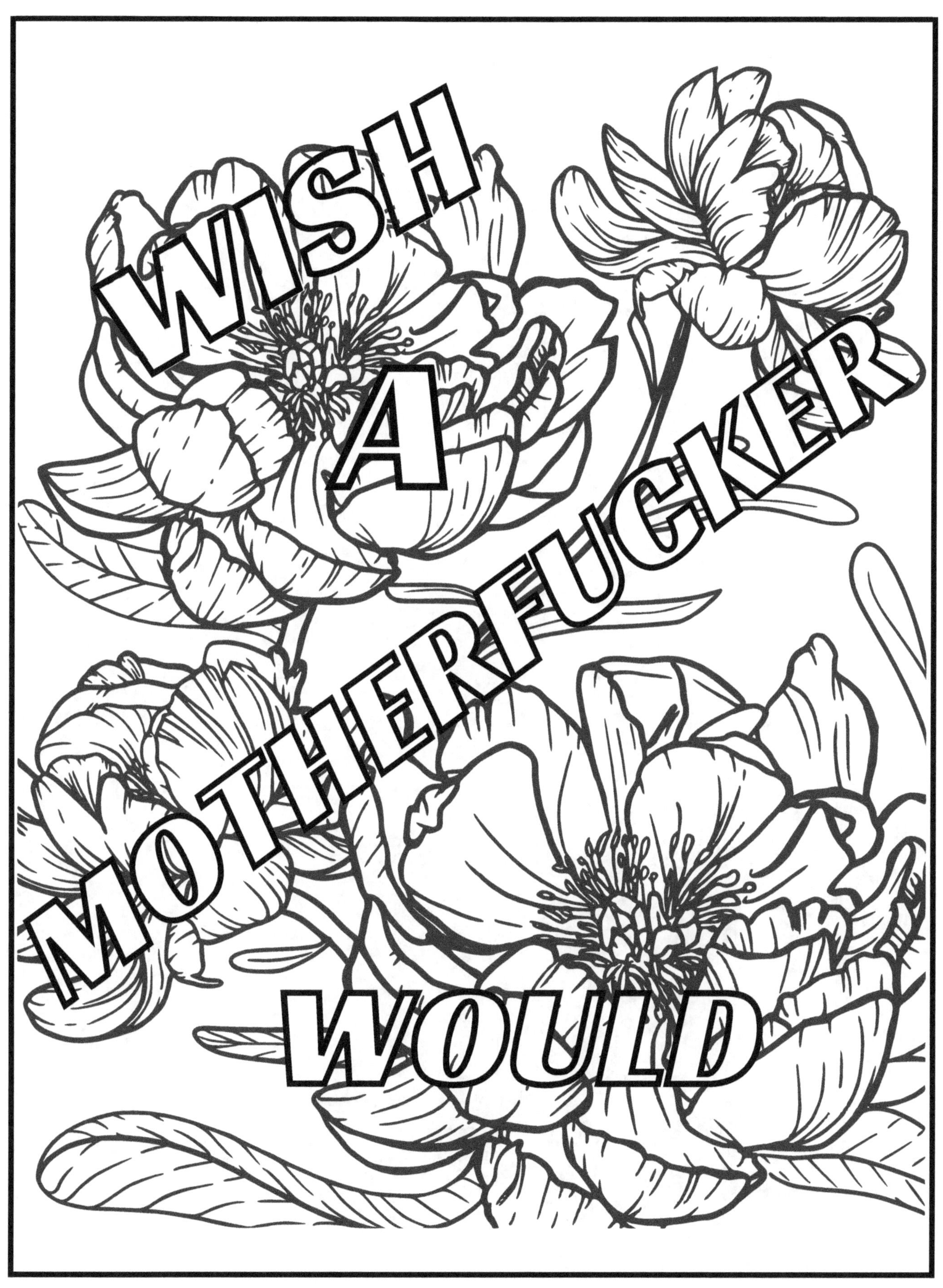

WISH
A
MOTHERFUCKER
WOULD

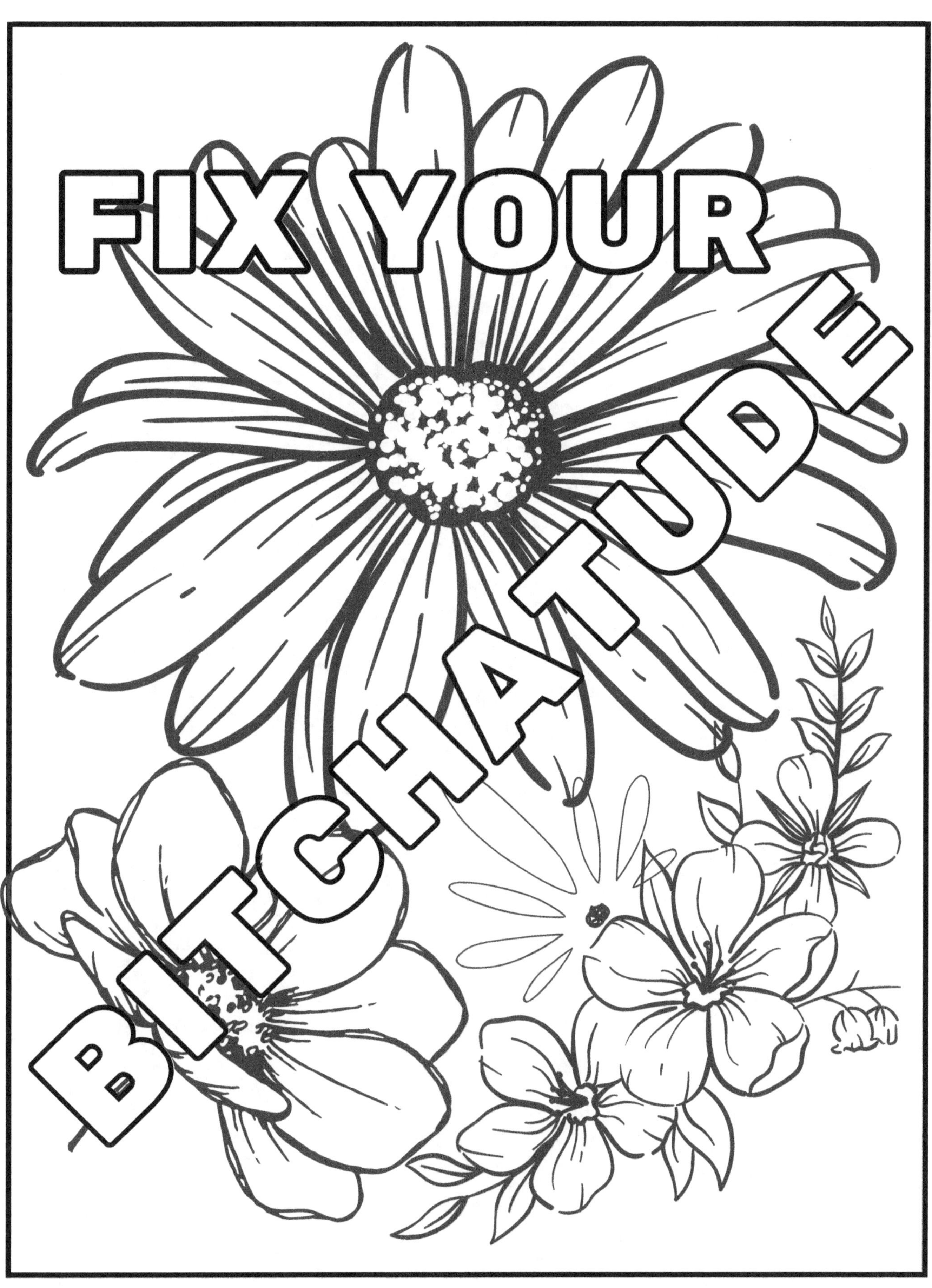

FIX YOUR
BITCHATUDE

FUCKERY
TWAT WAFFLE
ASSMUNCH
BITCHITIS
HOLY FUCK BALLS
SUCK NUTS
FTDS

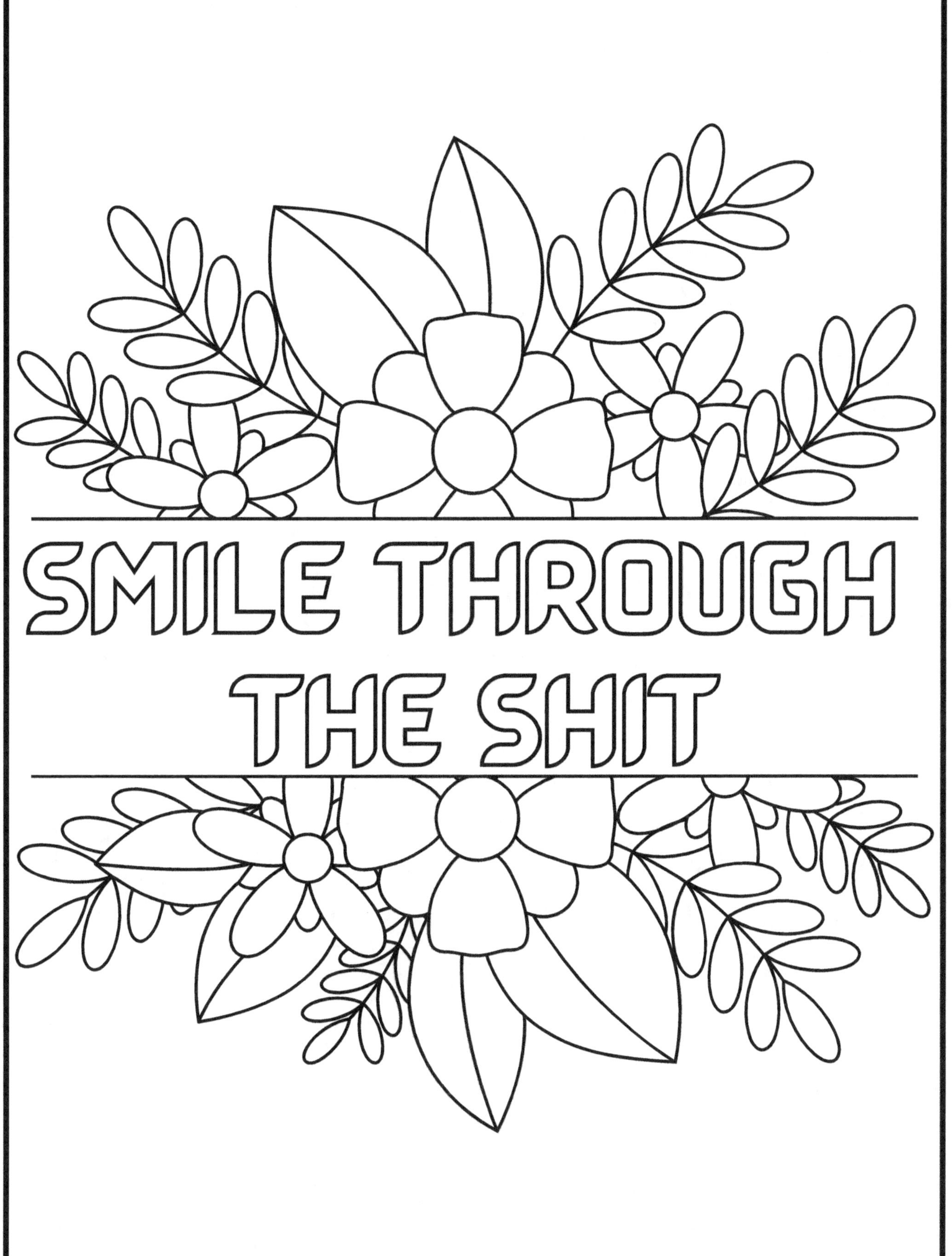

SMILE THROUGH
THE SHIT

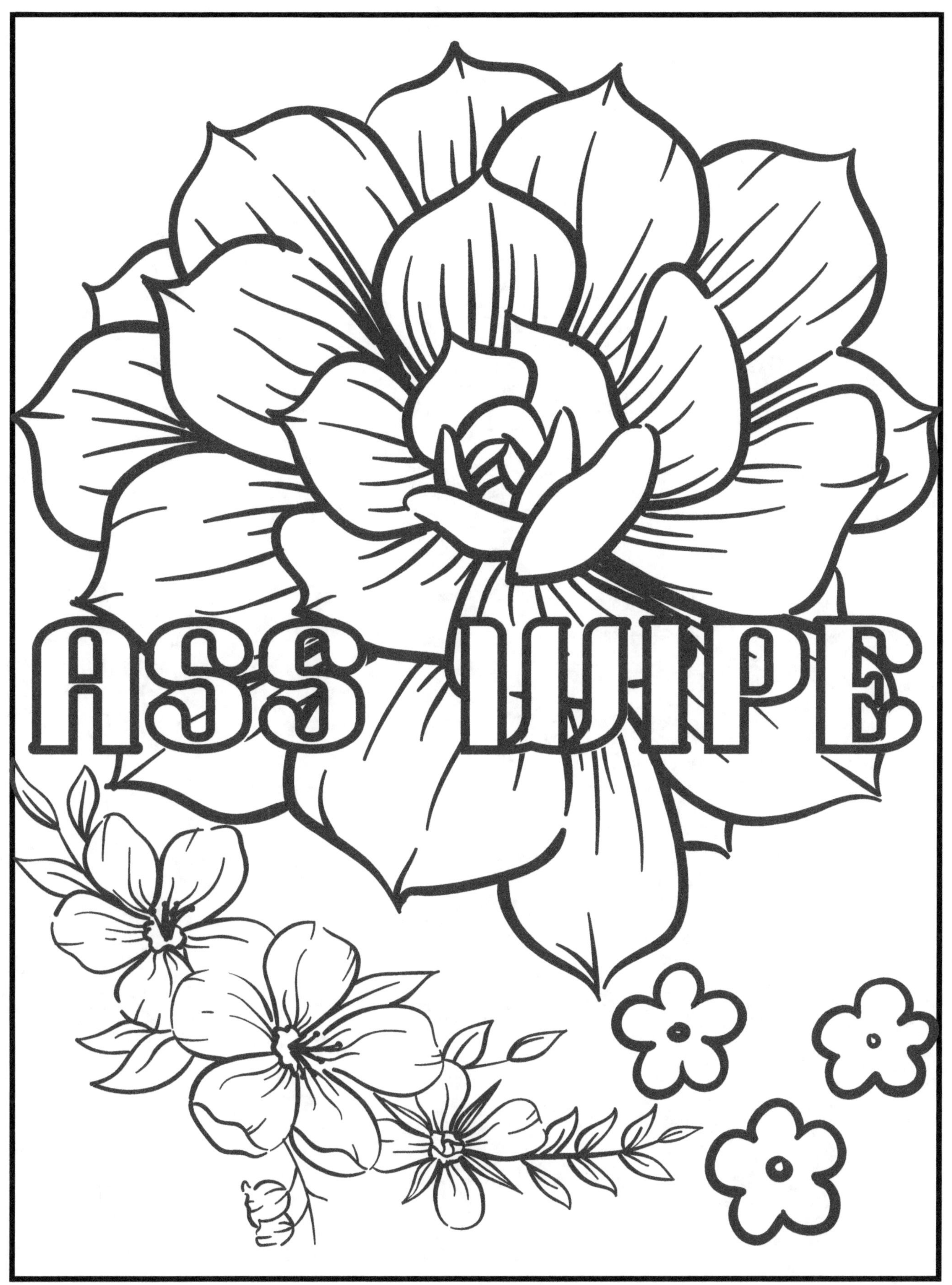
ASS WIPE

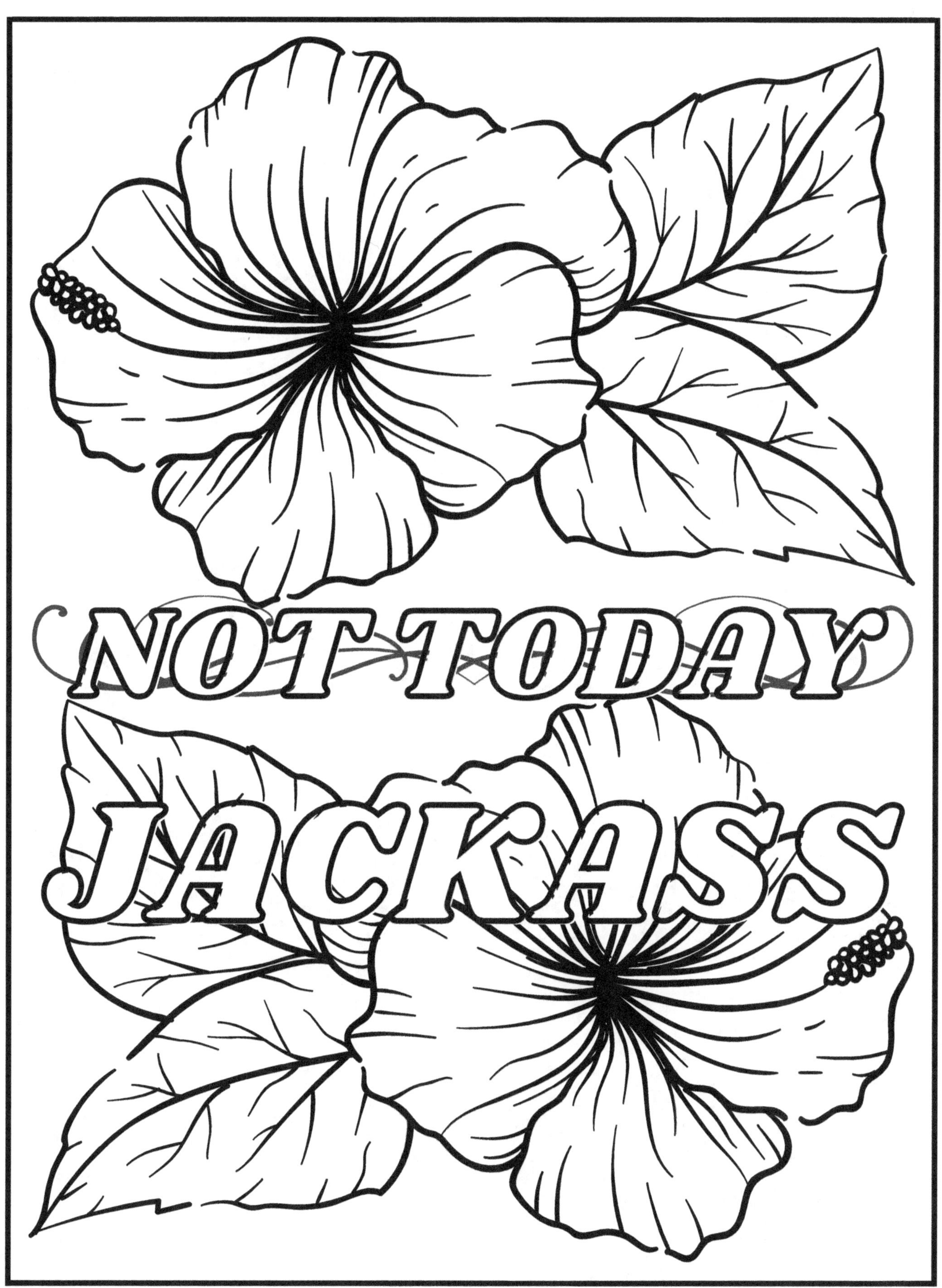

NOT TODAY
JACKASS

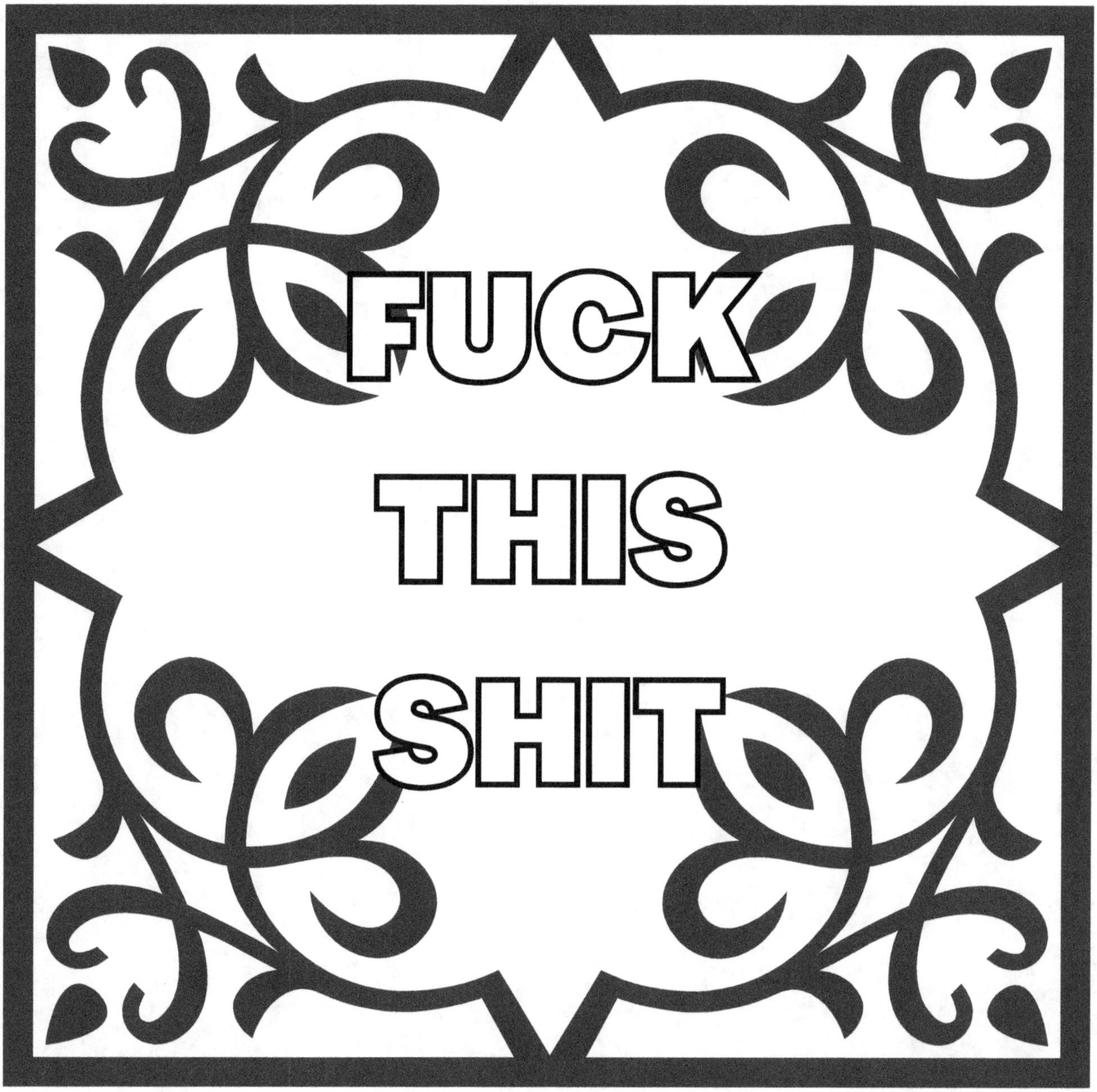

FUCK THIS SHIT

YOUR FAVORITE FUCKEN WORD

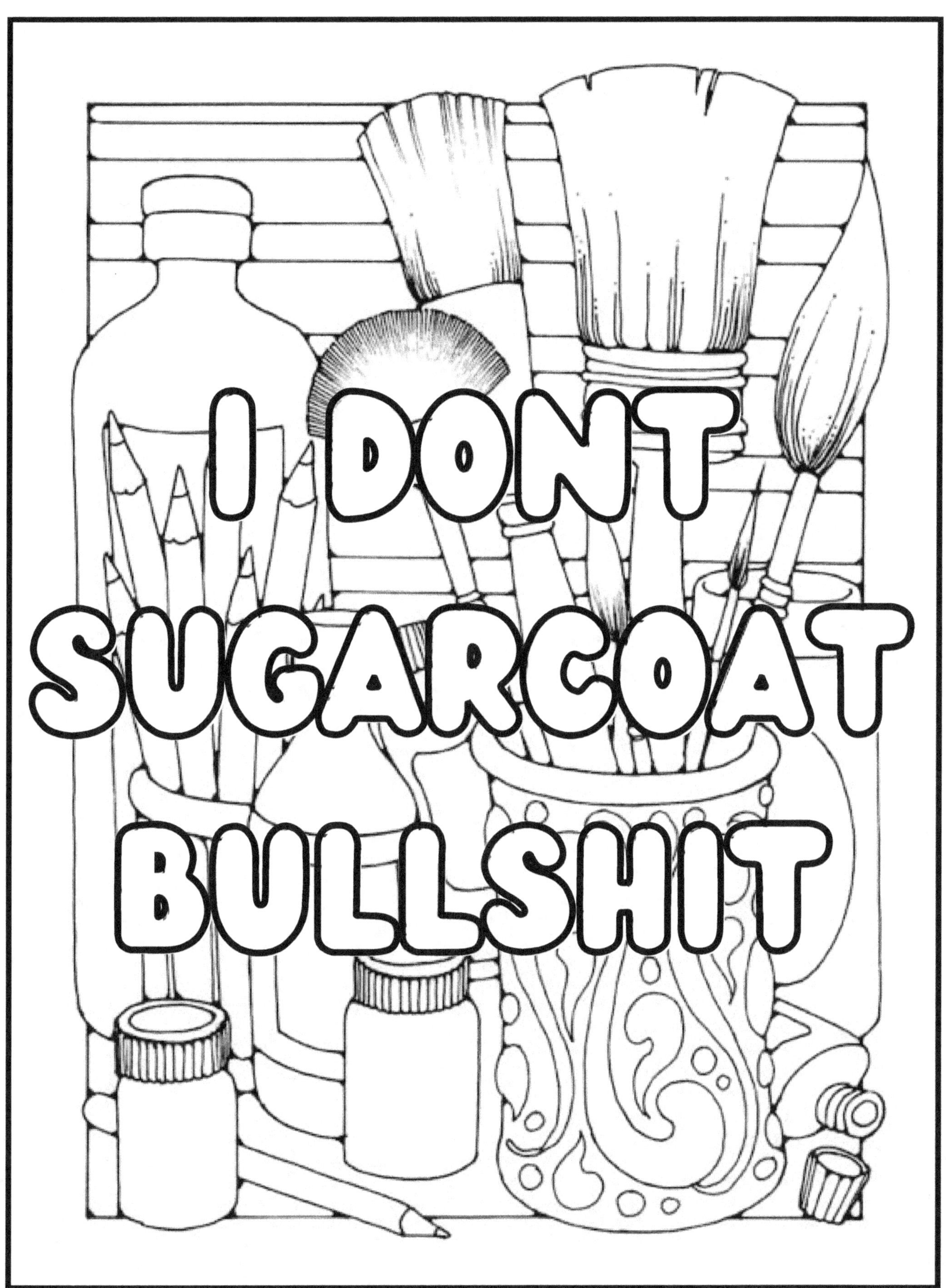

I DONT
SUGARCOAT
BULLSHIT

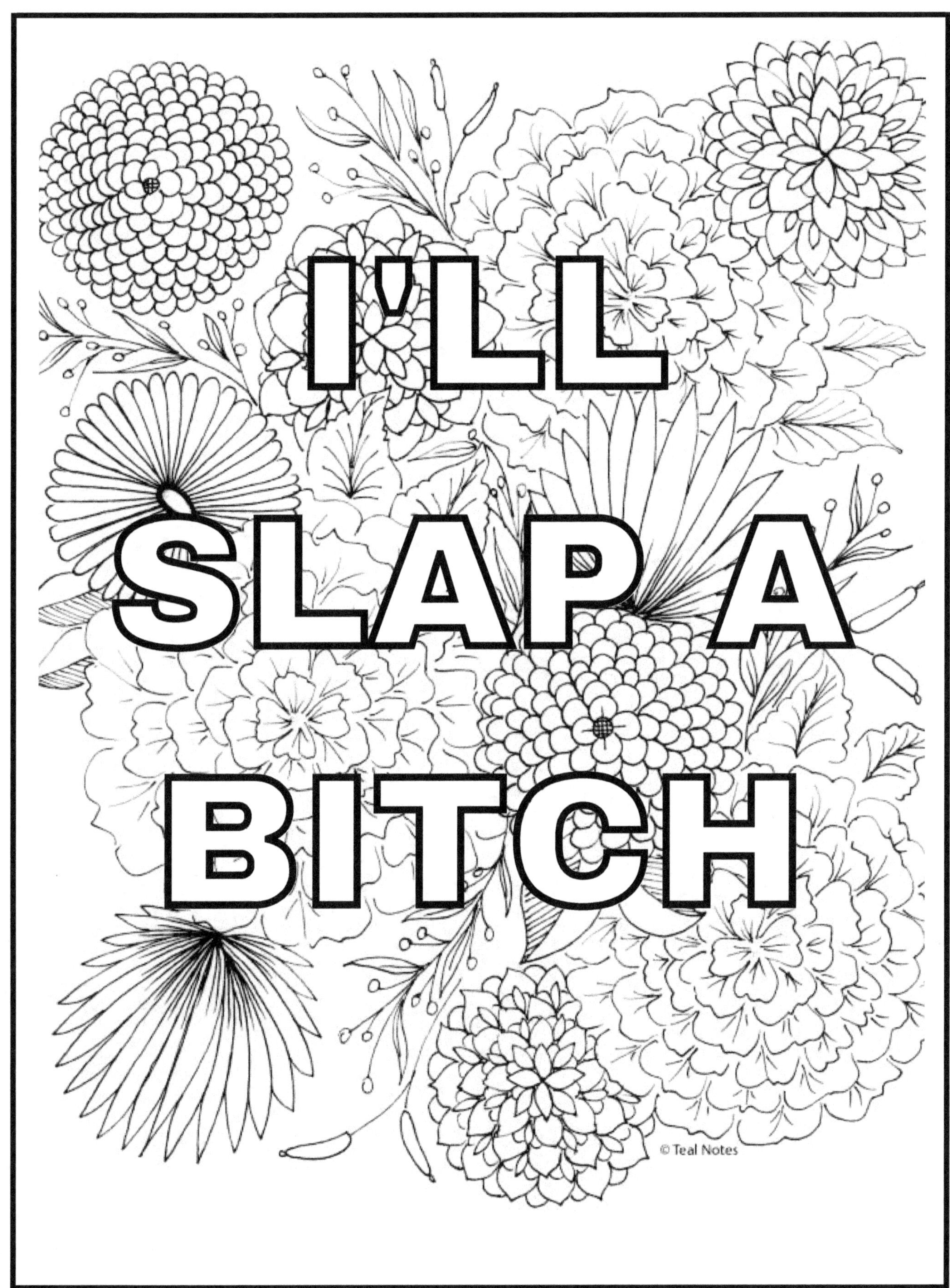
I'LL
SLAP A
BITCH
© Teal Notes

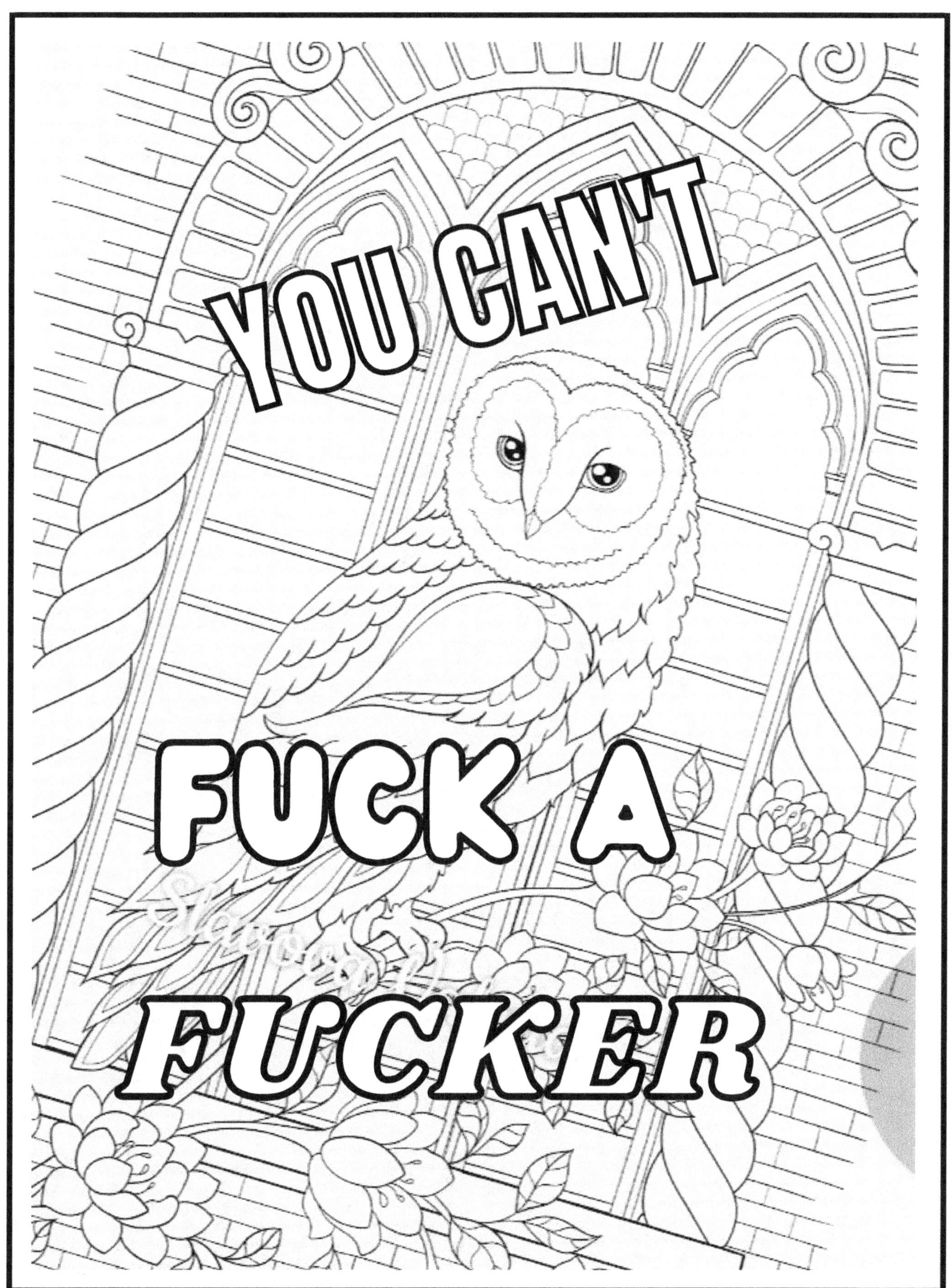
YOU CAN'T
FUCK A
FUCKER

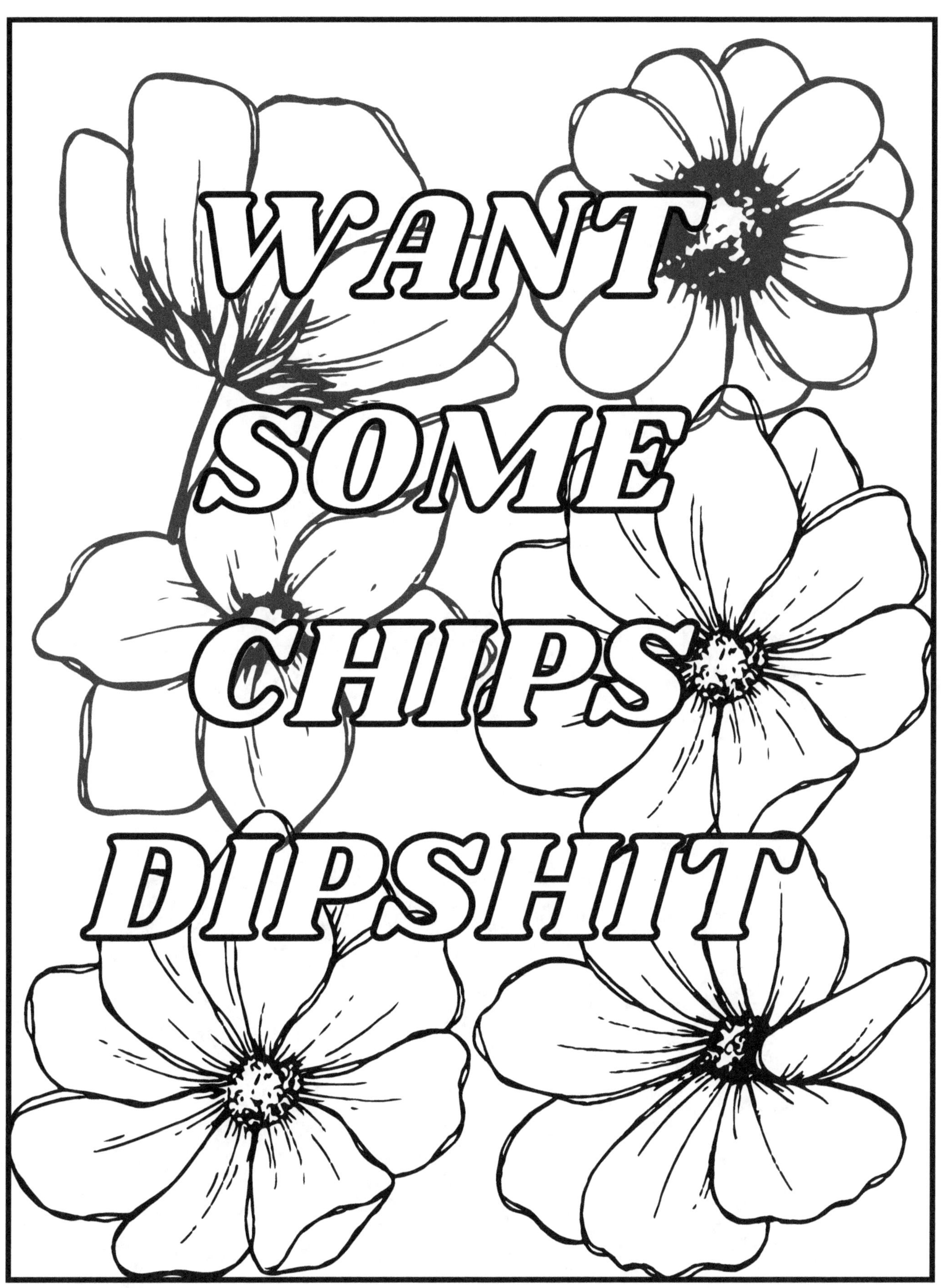

WANT
SOME
CHIPS
DIPSHIT

HOPE YOU
HAVE HAD A
GREAT DAMN
TIME.
RELAX UNWIND
ALWAYS BE
KIND